MW01482526

the sun will shine

the sun will shine

"Laura's kindness, fierce determination and strong-mindedness have undoubtedly shaped my outlook in life. Through her tenacity, Laura showed everyone around her how to persevere and accomplish every goal they set."
- TANYA BERG, FRIEND

"The questions everyone reading this book should ask themselves are: 'What do I want to be remembered for? What do I want my legacy to be?'"
- ROB HYNDMAN, FRIEND

"She was wiser at sixteen than any of us will ever be. Not many people at such a young age can leave such a profound mark on people's lives, on this community." **- NADIA COSTANZO, FRIEND**

"Like any other teenager she was embarrassed and was insecure about her disease and that she was different. She would get frustrated about not being able to use her body the way "normal" people would. But deep down she was like everyone else…she wanted to be included and had all of the usual insecurities a teenage girl has. She struggled

with the "why me" but also lived gracefully her entire life with dignity."
- CRISTINA BORGOGELLI, FRIEND

"Laura fought this insidious disease for a decade before finally succumbing to its deathly grip but during those 10 years the seeds of hope that she planted have grown in to massive Redwoods."
- GARY BEECH, RADIO PERSONALITY

"She possessed and passed on the traits that you would hope your children would own – selflessness, caring, thoughtfulness, bravery and leadership – all traits of real leaders in life." **- RICK GIOMMI, FRIEND**

"She consoled others when they wanted to console her... always saying, 'Don't worry, It's going to be okay'." **- SABRINA ROCCA, FRIEND**

"I have never met anyone like Laura and never will. I adored her passion to help others. It motivated me in life to be the best version of myself."
- CLAUDIA MANONI, FRIEND

the sun will shine

Laura Cotesta

Edited By Laura Stradiotto

StoriaBooks

Library and Archives Canada Cataloguing in Publication

Cotesta, Laura, 1978-1997, author
The sun will shine / Laura Cotesta ;
edited by Laura Stradiotto.

ISBN 978-1-988989-11-2 (softcover)

1. Cotesta, Laura, 1978-1997. 2. Cancer patients' writings.
3. Cancer--Patients--Canada--Biography. I. Stradiotto, Laura,
1978-, editor II. Title.

RC265.6.C67A3 2018   362.19699'40092   C2018-905796-3

Book design: Prajna Gandhi
Cover artwork: Cristina Borgogelli
Interior illustrations: Laura Cotesta

Published by: StoriaBooks
an imprint of Latitude 46 Publishing

109 Elm Street, Suite 205
Sudbury, Ontario P3C 1T4
info@latitude46publishing.com

Sometimes I think of writing a book about my story…maybe when my life settles down, I will find the time.

LAURA COTESTA

May 17, 1995

CONTENTS

FOREWARD

. . . .

On December 30, 1978 at 7:35 p.m. I became
a mother for the first time. There was an
overwhelming and over-joyous feeling of love that
struck me the moment I first held my precious little
baby and felt her take her first breath against my
heart.

On July 22, 1997 shortly after midnight, there was
a feeling of helplessness, and I was overcome with
sadness as I held my precious child for the last time
and felt her take her last breath against my heart.

The darkness and emptiness that I felt is
indescribable, but the life Laura lived in between her
first and last breath is what I wish to share with you
in this book.

This is Laura's journey.

Laura Cristina Cotesta was a cute, adorable child. So petite and dainty and always with a big smile on her face. I enjoyed every milestone with pride. Her first steps, her first words, her first day of school and her first ride on the big yellow bus. My heart was beating so hard, I will never forget letting her go for the first time. She was so proud of riding the bus all alone.

Her kindergarten teacher praised her; she was her little helper and she made friends with everyone in the class. Her smile was contagious and remains part of all her classmates' memory of her.

Life was great. We had just had our third child, purchased a new house and were in the prime of our lives. We were fortunate to have a large extended family always around us. Laura loved her two little sisters and was like their second mom. They were her pride and joy and in grade two, she made her first attempt in storytelling. She took first prize for her speech about her sister Daniela. She told everyone how her sister brought joy to her and her family, even though she was noisy, always banging on pots and pans. Laura's writing, along with her great expressions, made that speech unforgettable.

That summer we took a family trip to Vancouver with some friends. We had the time of our lives. We visited the zoo and all the tourist attractions possible

in that beautiful city. We went to the largest
waterparks in Canada. Laura had so much fun with
her sister Melissa going up and down the slides,
playing in the water, running around and splashing
each other. In the midst of this wonder, something
happened. As Laura slid down one of the slides, she
screamed from the top of her lungs. She had
experienced a sharp pain in her back when she
landed in the water. We weren't too worried and
brushed off the situation as something that happens
in a waterpark. But Laura's pain continued for the
rest of the family vacation. She carried on like a
typical child during the day but couldn't fall asleep at
night because her legs hurt and she couldn't lie
down. We had walked so much during the day that
we thought the pain in her legs was normal after a
long day. We reassured her that everything would
be okay.

Our vacation was over and Laura didn't complain
again until one calm Sunday afternoon. We were
outside cutting the grass and the kids were playing.
Suddenly Laura started crying and screaming like
she had done at the waterpark in Vancouver. We
thought it odd because there was no reason why she
should be feeling pain in her back and legs. She was
in the comfort of her own home, playing like a
normal child. Again, we reassured her that

everything was okay. But we started to worry.

Over the next few days, Laura saw several doctors: we were told that she was having growing pains and that it would go away. We were also told Laura was suffering from a lack of parental attention because our focus was being spread across three children. The anxiety and uncertainty, along with a crying child who wasn't sleeping, was taking a toll on us all.

We were referred to the Hospital for Sick Children in Toronto. The doctor there expressed the urgency for an MRI. That became the first horrifying experience of many for Laura as the MRI machine malfunctioned just before her turn. She was in so much pain because she had to lie down for the test.

The next option was to have a myelogram done on her back. This procedure is more invasive as a needle is inserted into the spine with a radioactive liquid so x-rays and pictures can show what was happening in the spinal canal. Laura had to be admitted to SickKids in Toronto for this procedure. She was moved by stretcher to a little room in a back dark hallway. I was asked to stay at the end of the hall where there was a waiting area.

Laura was afraid and crying so loudly I could hear her from down the hallway, but I could not be there to console her. I sat waiting, pacing and then panicking when I heard Laura scream again so loudly it echoed down the hallway. That sound remains a vivid memory for me, to this day.

I could not stay in the waiting room any longer and ran toward Laura, storming into the room, even though I was prohibited to be there for the procedure. I embraced her, held her tight, consoled her and tried to convince her that everything was going to be okay. I told her I would never leave her again.

That test revealed Laura had cancer and needed immediate surgery on her spine for the resection of a spinal cord tumour. Over the next ten years, the tumor would return five more times, all along a different segment of her spine. Although bedridden and challenged with the results of spinal surgeries for extended periods of time, Laura carried on to live with normalcy. We gave each other strength and dealt with things as they came.

She continued in her sports in any way she could. School was important to her. She wanted to graduate with her friends, learn to drive and have a "normal" life.

She applied to university and was ready to plunge into adulthood. The countless treatments, tests and procedures were a mere inconvenience for her. But she was so thankful to everyone who played a role in helping her to meet her goals.

Everything she achieved was meaningful. She made everyone feel good; she was always smiling, accepting her challenges and living life with purpose. She used these challenges to make an impact in the lives of others.

Laura was also vocal when it came to sharing her life experiences. A few days before her passing, lying in the intensive care unit, unable to speak, see, or hear, she asked for her family and friends. The police and security monitored the waves of people entering the hospital to visit her. Her body was weak and frail but she managed to scribble messages for us on a clipboard to make us all feel at ease. She made sure all her t's were crossed and her i's were dotted in every aspect of her life. She told us not to be afraid. She thanked us for being her friend.

Her message to me left a similar lump in my heart as the day I put her on the big yellow bus on her first day of school. Only this time, my heart was pounding with anxiety and fear. I could not accept that I had to let her go, for the last time.

My eyes filled with tears as she squeezed my hand and scribbled on the clipboard.

Please don't be afraid mom. I am not giving up…I just don't want to suffer any more. Don't forget me.

It is impossible to forget her.

She remains part of our lives through memories and the awards given in her honour at The Copper Cliff Skating Club, The Ida Sauve Dance Studio, St. Teresa, Holy Cross and St. Francis elementary schools, St. Benedict Catholic Secondary School, Relay for Life's "Love and Friendship Team", and through Lockerby Composite School, and its annual Kids Caring for Kids Remembering Laura Cotesta Cancer Drive.

Laura also left us her journals and messages of wisdom.

This project is giving Laura the opportunity to complete her wish of someday writing a book about her experiences. It demonstrates how she was able find peace and tranquility throughout her illness.

This feisty girl made my heart race every day of her life. There was nothing ordinary about her life. She had a magic spark and she taught us all that we can achieve what our hearts tell us to do.

If you keep hoping and praying for sunshine, the sunshine is sure to come.

- PINA COTESTA

INTRODUCTION

* * * * * * * * * * * * * * * *

Twenty years had passed since Laura left us, and
I was preparing to celebrate the twentieth year of
Kids Caring for Kids Remembering Laura Cotesta
Cancer Drive. The number added up to forty and by
coincidence the thought of Laura turning forty felt
pretty nostalgic. Where had all this time gone when
it seemed that we had lost her only yesterday?

I realized that life was chasing me and there were
things that needed to be done. One of those actions
was to go through Laura's belongings. We had
moved three times since her passing and each time
we moved, I made a special place in our homes for
her. Her schoolwork, artwork and journals rested in
boxes, untouched. I never had the courage to go
through them, always procrastinating and thinking

there would be another day, perhaps a better time.

I was truly blessed when I was able to witness the birth of my grandchildren. For the first time in a long time I felt an overwhelming joy in my heart. Here was a new generation of our family being brought into this world. It felt so surreal, yet wonderful. At the same time, I realized how fortunate I was to see many generations of young people experience Lockerby's Cancer Drive, something that was near and dear to Laura's heart.

I embraced my fears and found the courage to say I can, just like Laura. It was up to me to share her life with many and so I opened those boxes and pulled out Laura's journals, artwork and schoolwork.

I first approached Ronda Lenti, who was Laura's English teacher when she wrote her final journals and asked her if she could help me go through them and find the resources needed to begin this book writing journey. Although she had dealt with the loss of her own child, she plunged into the project with as much enthusiasm and passion as I had. We have both found the courage to expose the darkest moments of our lives, yet found the sunshine in Laura's words.

I then approached Laura Stradiotto, one of Laura's friends who witnessed her struggle, and she too found excitement in sharing her friend's journey.

She began to transcribe Laura's writing and edited her words into manuscript format. She also gathered testimonials from Laura's friends, former teachers and students who participated in the annual cancer drive to better understand Laura's impact.

Laura's writing is presented in four chapters: Happiness, Change, Loss and Hope. These are the four phases of the Wheel of Life, a cycle which repeats itself throughout a person's lifetime. We see the themes as the perfect vehicle to deliver Laura's message.

WHEEL OF LIFE

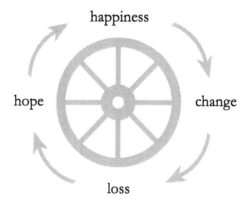

Laura's writing spans ten years and will appear mostly in chronological order, starting from the tender age of eight to the moments before she passed away at eighteen. Laura reflects on her life experiences throughout the book, often returning and re-evaluating the past with maturity and further insight.

In her journals and schoolwork, Laura expressed a desire to write a book. She even started writing chapters and would revisit them year after year, adding more detail as time passed.

This is her story. In her own words.

- PINA COTESTA

happiness

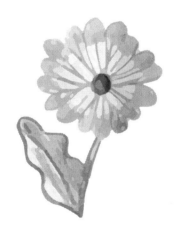

The Falling Star

I saw a falling star that filled the sky.
I was wondering what it was doing.
Mamma said it must be a star.

The Northern Lights

They are found in the north half of the world.
Although they start out as small flickers of light,
they can grow and grow.

Hail

One night there was a hail storm.
And the hail was the size of a baseball.
My sister was crying and it was noisy.

The Rainbow

Sometimes, right after it rains, the sun shines.
Then you may see a rainbow in the sky.

It's a good day.

Practice at the arena at 8:00.
We had a few falls but it is okay.
When we got home my mommy turned on
the electric curlers.

At Brownie's the group made a piggy purse.
Linda, Lindsay's mother said next week we
are going to get the arts and craft badge.

At dancing we learned a new step:
step-shuffle-step-step.
And we learned one more step:
shuffle-hop-shuffle-hop.
We practiced and practiced.

Today for gym we went sliding.
It was fun on that steep hill.

Guess what? I got straights A's.
I just knew I could do it! I just knew it!
I am very glad about that.

My Sister Daniela

She's special, she's a bundle of joy, she's cute, she is my sister Daniela.

"What are we going to call this new member of the family?" Daddy, Mommy, Melissa and I asked ourselves. Are we going to call her Paminina, Georgette or Mimi? I think none of these. Would you pick any of them? The family was so confused. One night the family decided that we would pick names out of my daddy's working hat. Out came Daniela. The family had a little fight because I wanted to call her Pamela. But then my mommy said, "We are going to call her Daniela." It was all right with me. But I was a little disappointed.

Now we are all over that, but not the crying. All we hear all day is waa, waa, waa. I am not complaining because we all did it too. And before I knew it, Daniela was crawling all over.

Guess what? Daniela is in the cupboards now! Cling, cling, cling, the clattering of pots and pans clinging together. The baby grew up fast. It's already Daniela's birthday. When I woke up I saw a little girl moving in the room. Who is it? Of course, it is Daniela. I should have known it!

When Daniela saw her birthday cake, she stuck her hand in the cake.

Mommy did not get there in time, so Daniela wipes her face with her hand. She looked funny! But she was full of icing. We took a picture quick, quick, quick.

Does anyone have an idea why Daniela has blue eyes and blonde hair? That's a mystery.

Do you know what Daniela calls herself? She calls herself DinDin.

She's special, she's a bundle of joy, she's cute, she's my sister Daniela.

Dear God,

I love you very much for
making our beautiful world.
I love you too for helping me
discover the world even more.
I thank you for making me a
family that loves me and cares
for me, that they too helped me
discover the ocean, the boats,
and told me not to be afraid.

At skating I did my first flip.
Amazing! Real amazing.

Summer Discoveries

When we went to Vancouver along with my
dad's friend, we went to the ocean. When we
were there the ocean was calm, but boy was it
cold! So, I asked my mom why the ocean was
so calm on a cold day. My mom said,
"Depending on where you are, the ocean is
either calm or rough, cold or windy."
This made me happy because now I am
interested in science.

Another thing I discovered while I was in
Vancouver was that you could put your car in
the ferry and travel from Vancouver to
Vancouver Island. This made me happy
because now I know a different way to travel.

My last discovery are the machines used to do
the Cat Scan on my back. They were big with a
lot of buttons. The big machines sure are
scary. I discovered these big machines are able
to take pictures of the bones, and only the
bones in my back.

T tulips, today, trees and teacher
H hugs, hill, hearts, houses and helicopters
A apples, animals, Arctic
N Nonno, Nonna, nose and numbers
K kisses, kings and kites
F fathers, friends, families and fish
U us, unicorns
L love, ladies, legs, life.

My values:

· To treat others as I would want to be treated
· To be kind to others
· To make full use of my potential and capabilities
· To be accepted
· To show self-control
· To make my own decisions
· To understand myself and others
· To be easy to get along with
· To show good judgement
· To be honest
· To work hard towards my goals
· To be dependable
· To share
· To be brave
· To be happy
· To get things I enjoy the most.

One of my happiest times was when I
came out of surgery and came home alive.

Queen of the Ice

Right now, if I could be anywhere, I would be flying through the air and landing my triple axel at the Olympics. I would be skating the performance of my life in a beautiful crimson and gold puffy sleeved dress. Kurt Browning at my side as he cheers me on, knowing I am going for the gold. Kristi Yamaguchi waiting, wondering and hoping she can beat me. As I land my quadruple toe she knows I am the winner and the one who is going to have the Olympic gold around my neck in the next half hour.

As I glide off the ice, Kurt sweeps me off my feet and hands me a bouquet of roses. As I wait for my marks, I have straight 6's across the screens as the Olympic gold is put around my neck and I become the Queen of the Ice at the age of thirteen!

Kurt Browning

Kurt Browning is his name,
in Alberta he was born and raised.
At Royal Glenora skating is his game,
and by his friends he is praised.

He won his first title,
in Chicoutimi Quebec.
Concentration is vital,
because he does not know what to expect.

A flip, a jump twirling high off the ice,
a quadruple he lands.
He makes it nice,
as the audience clap their hands.

To Germany, France and Spain he did go,
with Coach Jiranek by his side.
He has been World and Canadian Champion
Three times in a row,
and he is Canada's joy and pride.

A World Champion he continues to be,
in the Guinness Book his achievements have
been recorded.
With jumps, and loops and axels to see,
his quadruple will never be retorted.

Now that he is twenty-four,
and a man of five foot seven,
he will slowly close the door,
but he will always stand a winner in his
high heaven.

The Word That Means The World To Me

M is for the million things she gave me.
O means she's only growing old.
T is for the tears she shed to save me.
H is for her heart of purest gold.
E is for her eyes of love shining.
R means right and right she'll always be.

Mothers always want what's best for you; they protect you, they comfort you, they give of themselves to fulfill the needs of others. A special bond of love exists between a mother and her child.

My mother, Mrs. Giuseppina Cotesta, wanted what was best for me when she brought me to the Toronto Hospital for Sick Children to find out what was wrong with me. She protected me from all the doctors and nurses making sure they did not hurt me.

My mother comforted me when I was undergoing radiation treatment; she assured me everything would be fine. She gave of herself to fulfill my needs when she never left my side for three months.

My mother put her life on hold to stay with me in Toronto for three months and I will never forget that. We grew very close through that experience and through many others. Sometimes we say the same things and worry about the same things. Even though we have some differences, I believe that our relationship is very strong and unbreakable.

A special bond of love exists between my mother and me. Because of her dedication and persistence to keep me alive, I'm here today. One day I wish to save her life just as she saved mine.

The three most important things to know
in life are:

1. Who you are and who you want to be.
2. What your goal is in life.
3. That you are loved by your family
and friends.

To learn these things, we should cherish
and enjoy life.

We should always try our hardest to do
everything we do and be kind and loving
to our family and friends.

You should have a plan for your life and
understand your limits.

Our emotions help us express how
we feel inside.

When we have negative feelings, the
best thing to do is think positive and
hope for the best because if you
keep hoping and praying for the
best, it will come sometime.

The best feeling I've ever had is the
feeling of accomplishment, great
relief and happiness when I came
out of the hospital alive and three
years later, was Skater of the Year in
1989. Since then, I have been able to
gain my ability to skate.

Health is like a gift of life.

Strong faith and good health can get you
through anything.

Our bodies can help us to get in touch
with God because if we use our bodies to
do good things, we are following in Jesus'
footsteps and trying to be a good person.
Nobody has a perfect body but we can all
respect our bodies and the bodies of
others and everyone can try and respect
and take care of how our bodies grow.

If we learn to make good decisions now we will continue to make good decisions throughout life and be responsible.

The three most important decisions a person makes in life is:
1. to follow their faith,
2. their guidance and career
3. who they are going to marry.

The hardest thing to decide when you are a follower of Jesus is whether to believe and follow in Jesus' footsteps or to turn your back on him.

Young people can help the world
to be a better place by trying to be
the best person they know how to
be, always telling the truth, trying
their hardest in everything and by
always having faith in God.

Death is a part of life that tests our
faith, tests how we live and how much
we love our life.

I believe that after we die, we start a
new life with God that is better and
happier than the life we live on earth.

The most complete person we will be is
the person we are when we die because
we have already lived the best life we
could possibly live.

If it is your time to die, you must. God
probably needs your love up in heaven.

change

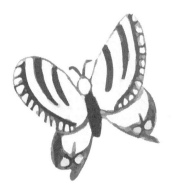

A raging storm is often an unexpected occurrence. In the distance we hear it rage and feel that it will pass – go around us – not disrupt our plans or routine. When the great storm strikes and blows you off your feet, we are forced to re-evaluate our priorities, weigh our plans, let go and ignore what things seemed so important before the terrible storm. Building from scratch, it rages, threatens, frightens and bewilders. Then one day when we least expect it, it disappears. After this the sun covers the storm and shines brighter than we've ever known it to shine.

Spring Newness

As the flowers start to bloom,
and the trees start to bud,
caterpillars spin cocoons,
and the earth turns to mud.

The birds sing in harmony,
like a choir,
with their colony,
until they tire.

The earth is high and low,
and the snow disappears.
The green grass starts to grow,
and the trees reappear.

As the thunderous clouds rain down on us,
Spring is a time for newness.

I was the 81st child in the world to have
an ependymoma spinal cord tumour.

> I was in the hospital for two months
> because I had a spinal cord tumour.
> A tumour is something like cancer,
> but it's not quite like cancer because a
> tumour can only come in one place and
> cancer can spread all over your body.
> That's why I should be thankful, that I
> got a tumour in my spinal cord and not
> in my brain.

What would make me happy is if
my hair could just sprout out,
just if I put water on it like a flower.
If my hair grew like that I would be
happy because I HATE my wig.

Another thing that would make me
happy is if nobody in the world would
ever get cancer because it's very
painful to go through.

At one point in life everyone experiences
some pain and sorrow.

It all started one beautiful evening in Vancouver
B.C., the last night of a marvellous vacation. It was
bedtime when I felt tremendous pain raging in my
upper thighs and buttocks. My parents checked me
thoroughly and since there was nothing visible, they
just replied, "Oh! It's nothing. You're only growing."

When my family and I reached home the pain just
kept shooting down my thighs. Everyone thought
there was something wrong. But what? The family
doctor said to take aspirin for pain.

A week passed and the pain got so irresistible that
it was terribly hard to sleep, walk, lie down or sit.
No one could figure out what was wrong. Everyone
gasped, "It's such a strange situation."

I was taken to see a pediatrician in Sudbury.
He took a look at me and said nothing was wrong.
I looked healthy and answered all his questions
intelligently. He touched the area where the pain was
and like a magical trick, I felt no more pain. At this
time, he turned around and bluntly expressed his

feelings to my parents. "There's nothing wrong with this child," he said. "I feel she is trying to get a message through to the people around her. It appears she wants attention and expresses it in this make-believe pain. She suffers psychologically and nothing more than that!"

His opinion was surely wrong! My pain was a true pain but why didn't he believe me? I felt so alone. My parents felt what 'Dr. Magic Touch' had shouted was certainly wrong. We went to see our family doctor again. He referred us to a nerve specialist, later a bone specialist and the list goes on.

The pain kept raging through me. I hoped it would pass but it did not.

I was brought down to the Toronto Hospital for Sick Children. Luckily, there we found Dr. Harold Hoffman. Dr. Hoffman checked me thoroughly. He then took a prickly wheel and rolled it along my left foot and then along my right. He looked at my parents and with hope said, "It seems your child has a problem in her lower back. There is some kind of pressure causing her to have lost feeling in her right foot. The pressure is unknown and requires further investigation." An MRI scan was immediately scheduled.

The MRI scan itself was a horrifying situation. Despite the fact that the machine broke down when it was my turn, I couldn't even lie still when repaired.

My mother and I were all alone in a gigantic city, frightened that no one would be able to discover the cause of this dreadful pain. After plenty of persistence, the worst happened. I had been diagnosed with a malignant spinal cord tumour. This is a very rare type of cancer in children.

Like a big storm my family was struck and blown off their feet. We were all forced to re-evaluate our lives and change our plans. In my heart, I knew my life would never be the same.

Surgery had to be performed. I knew it would be a very painful recovery. But unfortunately, the recovery was not the only hurdle I had to jump. I had to go through radiation therapy and suffer the consequences of this treatment.

My life had been threatened and I was frightened and bewildered to why all these unexpected things were happening to me. After all, I was only eight years old and suddenly I could no longer enjoy the normal childhood I was expected to. No more friends, dancing, skating, school nor family around me.

Two months later I came back home, to my family and friends.

One thing I learned through this experience is that there's always sunshine after a great storm. No matter how rotten you think something is, if you keep hoping and praying for the sunshine, the sunshine is sure to come.

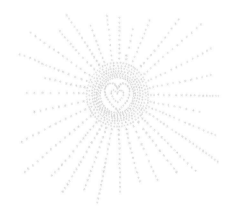

Cancer is a disease in which our cells grow
abnormally in some organ or tissue.

These cells go out of control, grow and increase in
number. Normal cells renew themselves throughout
life, but in an orderly and controlled manner. Normal
growth occurs when worn out tissues are replaced
and wounds heal. When cells grow out of control,
they form a mass and clump together. This is called
a tumour.

Some tumours become big where they begin to grow
and these are called benign tumours. Other tumours
not only enlarge locally but also can spread and
destroy the normal tissue around and go to other
parts of the body. Such tumours are called malignant
tumours, or cancer.

A spread of cancer occurs when malignant cells
separate themselves from the original tumour and are
carried to other parts of the body. Cancer can be
treated by chemotherapy and radiotherapy.
Chemotherapy is a treatment with anti-cancer drugs,
that are very effective on this type of disease.
Chemotherapy has a lot of side effects like nausea,
vomiting, diarrhea, hair loss, anemia, bleeding and

infections. Radiotherapy has pretty much the same side effects as chemotherapy.

Just recently I got sick with a tumour. I had radiotherapy treatment done to my central nervous system. I hope no one ever gets sick like I did, but we all know that cancer is a part of our life. I hope that doctors can find a cure for the disease so people do not have to suffer.

Why me, why me? Why do I have to get a brace for my back? I probably won't be able to do anything with it on. I have to wear it twenty hours a day. It takes two months to make. When they were measuring it on me, I turned blue and purple. I hope I'll be okay with the horrible brace. But it's better than surgery again.

One day I hope to write a book and star
in my own movie of my horror story.
I would tell the world how lucky I am to
be alive and to live your life to the fullest.

My number one fear in the world is to get
sick again. I am also afraid of one day
being known as the mean girl. I hate
knowing that people don't like me, and I
don't like knowing that some people are
scared of catching what I had.

I think that I am mean, nosy, bossy and
impatient sometimes and other times I
can be kind in helping people and caring,
loving and comforting them too.

My interests are skating, dancing, skiing
and swimming. My greatest loves are my
family and especially my mom who saved
my life and is a living angel.

My Story - A Six Chapter Reflection

Chapter One: The First Occurrence

On July 31, 1987, I was cutting the lawn with my
dad when I had to stop immediately because of
some kind of strange pain in my thighs.
I complained about this discomfort to my dad.
He advised me to go inside for a rest. I followed
his instructions.

A week later while preparing for our family trip to
Vancouver, British Columbia, I felt the pain again.
I told no one. While sleeping that night the pain
struck me again. I awoke abruptly. During that
period, I prayed to God to make this unwanted pain
disappear. When morning came, I awakened
painless. God had answered my prayer. Had my
pain disappeared forever?

Chapter Two: Going West

No, my horror story had just begun. After two
nights in Vancouver, the pain started again.
This time it really hurt, it struck my upper thighs
randomly. Like lightning bolts, it shot up my thighs
and into my buttocks.

Why was this happening to me? I cried and for the first time I told my parents. My parents encouraged me not to think about it and go back to sleep. That night the pain left me. But for how long?

Chapter Three: Searching For An Answer

A week after we returned from Vancouver, the pain struck again. But this time it was greater. For the second time I complained to my parents. My parents did everything they could to help the pain disappear. They searched for an answer through sleepless nights. There was nothing they could do except keep hoping and praying. My parents did what was best and brought me to see our family doctor. He found nothing wrong and told my parents that it was just growing pains and all he could say was to take extra strength aspirin and stay in bed until the pain disappeared. We did as he advised but by the next week, we were back where we started, in his office with no answers and no cure. But when the doctor checked me over, he found something wrong, but still no answer. What he did do was refer us to the pediatrician in Sudbury.

When we got to his office we were called right in.

As we walked in, he impatiently told me to get undressed. At once he bluntly ordered me to touch my toes. I tried and tried but still I couldn't. He forced me to continue this movement until I finally did. After he touched the area where the pain was, the pain disappeared like magic. At this he turned around and bluntly expressed his feelings at my parents, "There is nothing wrong with this child! I feel that she is trying to get a message through to the people around her. It appears she wants attention and is expressing it in this make-believe pain! She suffers psychologically and nothing more than that!"

As I listened to these words, I could not comprehend what they meant. These words left my mother in astonishment. She swiftly turned around, grabbed my hand and immediately walked out the door angrily. While in the car I questioned my mother repeatedly. But she wouldn't answer. Was what the doctor told my mother serious?

Chapter Four: Please, Let Them Be Wrong!

Unfortunately, it was. The night while going to bed I felt inquisitive again and started to question my

mother. As I persisted in my questioning, my
mother sat on my bed with a tear rolling down her
cheek and she asked me, "Laura, are you faking the
pain because you don't want to go to school or
because you want attention?"

In anger, I threw myself on my bed, my face red in
horror. At once, I started to shout boisterously at
my mother, "How can you say that? I thought you
trusted me! I thought you believed me! I hate you
for thinking that!!!"

I walked out of my bedroom briskly and slammed
the door behind me. I went to a corner in the
hallway, hid my face and started to weep. My heart
was broken and I was terribly confused. "Why
doesn't anyone believe me? My legs do hurt!
It's true!"

A few minutes later my mom picked me up timidly
and replied, "Laura I'm sorry, I never meant to hurt
your feelings. Just that he's the best pediatrician in
Sudbury. And I want what's best for you. Tomorrow
I will call our family doctor again and go see him.
He will advise us as to who we can go see for a
second opinion. Oh Laura, I'm sorry."

The next day when we went to see the doctor, he was astonished with the news my mother told him. At once he made an appointment with another doctor. Day after day, I went from doctor to doctor with no answer. Just like broken records, they repeated what the other doctors had said.

Finally, after four weeks in pain, we went to see a neurosurgeon. After he checked me thoroughly he told my mother, sincerely, that I either had a herniated disk or a tumour. My mother understood, but I didn't for some strange reason. I felt that what the doctor had assumed was something horrible.

That night after telling my dad what happened, we decided to go visit my grandparents. As we walked in, my grandmother immediately started to ask my mother questions about what the doctor had said. As my mother explained about this tumour thing, she started to cry. I still did not understand, but I knew I was in trouble, something was terribly wrong.

Chapter Five: Little Did We Know

The next day we found ourselves back at our family

doctor's office. As my mother described to him what the neurosurgeon had thought the pain was, and that she still wanted another opinion, but not from a Sudbury doctor, but from a Toronto specialist. After much persistence from my mother, he finally agreed.

The next day my mom got a call from our family doctor telling her that he had made an appointment in Toronto at the Hospital For Sick Children with the head neurosurgeon in North America on Monday September 28 1987.

In two weeks I found myself painfully sitting in a crowded doctor's clinic. For four hours we waited to see Dr. Hoffman. We were called in and the nurse directed us to the room where he checked his patients. She then advised me to get undressed. A few minutes later Dr. Hoffman entered the room. He wasn't what I expected as a doctor at all. He was tall, skinny and wore glasses at the tip of his nose. He looked like a trustworthy doctor. At once he checked me thoroughly. He asked me questions about my pain. He advised me to touch my toes, but I couldn't. He then rolled a prickly wheel along my left foot and then along my right. I could see his movements but I couldn't feel them. I couldn't feel the prickly wheel on my right foot.

Dr. Hoffman turned around and with hope said, "It seems your child has a problem in her lower back. There is some kind of pressure causing here to have lost the feeling in her right foot. The pressure is unknown and requires further investigation."

An MRI scan was immediately scheduled for the next day. For hours we looked for a hotel. Finally, we found one. I guess it was half decent. My father didn't want to leave my mother and me all alone in Toronto but my mother finally convinced him into leaving us and she said that after the MRI scan we would take the bus home to Sudbury. We only prepared ourselves for one more day in Toronto but little did we know what was coming up.

Chapter 6: Persistence

The next day while waiting painfully for the MRI, the nurse came and told us the MRI scan (machine) had broken down. She explained that the piece needed for the machine to be fixed must come from the U.S. and might take until the next day at about

noon. My mother was furious. We had to stay in
Toronto longer with me in pain and nowhere to go.
The nurse told us to go to a place called the hostel
for people in limbo like us.

Noon came painfully. My mom and I found
ourselves in agony again at the MRI scan.
Unfortunately, the machine was not fixed. My
mother was persistent in that she wanted to help
me. We stayed nine hours in the stuffed up, warm,
sticky waiting room.

The nurses tried for hours to pass me through the
long tunnel but they had no luck. I was restless. I
could not stay still. They gave me a break. We called
my dad. My dad directed me to have confidence.
But there was too much pain. I could not fight it.
They tried again and again. No luck. We were then
sent to the hostel again.

The night was painfully uncomfortable and
annoying but I survived. The next day I found out I
was to have a 10-cm long needle injecting fluid into
my back. After a boisterous yell, it was over.

But as soon as they put me upside down, there was

something terribly wrong. The test did not work. There was something blocking the fluid from going down my spinal cord.

The doctors knew what was wrong. I had a spinal cord tumour. They had to do immediate surgery, but they did not have the information on how far up the tumour was, or what kind of tumour it was. I was put in the Hospital for Sick Children Ward G, 5th floor that night and watched like a hawk.

The next morning when I awoke, I was put to sleep. I was brought to have another MRI. This time it was successful. The doctors knew that I had ependymoma spinal cord tumour and that the tumour was five vertebrae up from my tail bone. For three days I was watched continuously.

Editor's note: Laura's journals contained multiple drafts of this story within a three year span. The story reprinted here represents her final draft.

Illness is probably harder for the caregiver to deal with than it is for the sufferer.

In my experience, I depend on my mom a lot and I think it's unfair for her to have to help me so much. But the medical system today wants to save money so they have to cut back nursing staff, funding for tests, funding for doctors and the list goes on. This puts tremendous pressure on the caregiver.

If I had an illness that would make me die,
I would want to be told AT ONCE.

· so I could continue to improve my faith,
· so I could have the sacrament of death,
· so I could finish living my life to the fullest,
· so I could say goodbye and I LOVE YOU
to all my family and friends.

After death I would like to be
remembered because:

· I was a great person.

· I loved my family and friends.

· I had a nice personality.

Me and Pain

There once was a girl who started to cry,
because she had great pain in her thighs.
For she could not walk, sit or stand,
because her pain was so grand.

Yet the doctors said,
it was all in her head.
But her mother believed,
that she could be relieved.

So, they went to Toronto,
very el pronto.
And there the doctors found,
that she had a mound.

In the back of her spine,
growing long like a grape vine,
she had cancer.
But the doctors had no answer.

So, after much panic,
and becoming ecstatic,
the girl had an operation,
and underwent radiation.

For she lost her hair,
and a wig she did wear.
For one day her cells did go crazy,
and she did become very lazy.

But she tried to cope,
and never ever lost hope;
that she would be alive,
and live a full life.

In 1989 she was skater of the year,
dispensing all her fear.
But now she has to wear a brace,
trying to show her face.

That is why she is here,
not having much fear.
To show the whole world,
who she is and what she's achieved.

I worship my hair more than the average person.

I think this is because of this fear I have of losing my hair again. When I was eight and I found out I was going to lose my hair, we cut my long, thick hair into a mushroom cut. I hated it and was unhappy for days.

We also had to buy a wig, and of course, the wig was short haired, too. I guess it was for the better because when my hair started falling out in clumps, I was devastated. It was better for me to go around with a short haired wig, that way as my hair grew back, I was able to take the wig off without a drastic change in hair length.

I think that being bald was one of the hardest things I had to deal with at the time. I know that hair plays an important role in everyone's life. Every morning we wake up and fix our hair. We need to have it right or we try again. Everyone's preference in hair length varies but I don't like anything shorter than chin length for myself. The short look is more sophisticated while longer hair is more childlike, but I think it depends on what you do with it, that defines your own image.

I think people should try to do the best they can with the hair they have, because you'll never know when it will be gone and you will want what you had back.

Change is good, but too much is bad.

Courage

She looks into the mirror,
almost every single day.
Looking at the exterior,
she surely looks okay.

Trying to find out
what's wrong inside,
is without a doubt
something she can't hide.

Nothing she feels
can be understood.
It doesn't seem real
or the way it should.

She must be brave,
for it will get brighter.
Every second she saves,
she becomes a strong fighter.

Being strong must be her goal.
She must find hope deep in her soul.
Fighting back unwanted tears,
from deep inside her strength appears.

I sometimes wonder what my life would be like if I had never gotten sick in the first place. What would I look like? What more could I have accomplished?

I was a good dancer, skater and swimmer. I was flexible and petite and always had fun. If nothing would have happened, I probably would be working as a lifeguard and skating coach and maybe still dancing. I would probably be on student council and part of the school more than I am now.

I almost feel like I was deprived of my childhood. Everything I had planned for myself was changed by illness. I always refer back to the things I could do then and forget about the things I can do now. I know that I almost died a number of times, but why can't I consider myself lucky?

Our society today refuses to accept fate or
what is meant to be.

We feel the need to control what happens and to
make it turn out the way we want it to.
Unfortunately, life isn't like that. Things happen
that are beyond our control and all we can do is
deal with them the best way possible.

Having had a very hard past three years, I know
what it means to be given a deck of cards,
without knowing how to deal with them.

I firmly believe that the paths we are forced to
take in life are chosen for us. The people who
deal with things the best are the ones who accept
the hurdle and jump over it.

I know there is nothing you can do to prevent
things from happening, but what I do know is
that you have to deal with things one day at a
time. All you can do is keep smiling and move on.

L'inconnu

On ne sait pas
ce qui va passer dans la vie.
On ne sait pas quand on va mourir,
et on ne sait pas quand on vit.
C'est l'inconnu.

On vit jour par jour,
mais on ne sait pas le future.
On a seulement l'espoir que Dieu
a choisi la même voie pour nous,
ce qu'on veut.
C'est l'inconnu.

Tous les soirs,
on dit une prière,
mais si Dieu va y répondre?
On ne sait pas,
C'est l'inconnu.

Si demain on va être mort,
Si demain le monde va se terminer,
Si demain notre vie va être changer
on ne sait pas,
C'est l'inconnu.

Dans notre voyage de la vie,
on espère tout,
mais ce que nous accomplirons
on ne sait pas,
C'est l'inconnu.

La futur du monde,
la guerre,
la malheur,
on ne sait pas,
C'est l'inconnu.

La santé,
les maladies,
les remèdes,
on ne sait pas,
C'est l'inconnu.

Les étoiles,
le ciel,
le soleil,
les autres planets,
on ne sait pas,
C'est l'inconnu.

On ne sait pas,
tout…..
C'est l'inconnu.

loss

· · · · · · · · · · · · · · · · ·

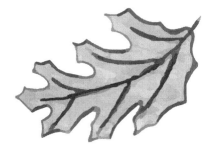

The news I received was unbelievable.

Dr. Hoffman gave me the results of the MRI Scan. He came toward us frowning, with his hands behind his back. I knew there was something wrong but had no idea what.

Dr. Hoffman told me that my tumour had come back and it had to be removed immediately. I almost started to cry but it didn't seem real. How could I be sick again? I've been fine for nearly six years. He showed us the scan and it was true.

The question of, "why me?" has been pounding in my head since the moment I found out. I hope I can keep my head on straight and my fears under control so this nightmare will not be as long as my last.

I feel like my life is happening on a TV screen, and I'm just sitting on the couch watching it progress.

I only found out Friday, and now I'm already in Toronto getting ready for surgery. It doesn't seem real. I have just left my life at home to face a new one. I don't know how long I will be here, but I hope it's not forty-two days like last time.

I am sitting here in this hospital bed wondering if my life will be drastically changed once I go to surgery tomorrow. I hope the anesthesiologist with the big nose doesn't put me to sleep tomorrow. He better let me pick the needle, because I definitely do not want the mask. The nurse that looks like a witch better not be mean to me, because now I am old enough to tell her how I feel.

I've taken my shower with the smelly soap, disinfected my back and been poked and pinched several times.

I think I am ready to have surgery but something is telling me that I should be afraid. My stomach has butterflies in it and I feel like I'm going to throw up. I am not scared of dying, but I am afraid of the short and long-term side effects this five-and-a-half-hour surgery will have on my life.

I know I can make it through this, I just have to be strong. I wished for everything to turn out right, on the first star I saw tonight.

I do not know how I will get to sleep, my heart is beating so hard it is about to pop out of my throat.

I wish a life without cancer could be
achieved as simply as taking an aspirin.

The thing I hate the most is the fact that I am
not a very healthy person.

Since the age of eight I have been in a constant
battle against cancer. I was so innocent and I did
not understand enough about life to have ever
guessed that I would be in this position today.

After six years of trying to forget my dreadful
experience, I was diagnosed with cancer again in
July 1993. I then underwent another five-hour
operation. I thought this would be the end of my
battle because I was told the tumour was taken
out. I got better over the three months that
followed but my recovery took a downfall when
I was diagnosed with cancer again on November
5th of 1993. That was followed by the news that
I must undergo radiation treatment again.

I am trying to recover from this nightmare.
I understand that I should be grateful that I am
alive and I have lived through two major
surgeries, two doses of radiation and all the bad
things that come with having cancer, but I have
yet to understand why God has chosen me to be
the one to suffer.

I don't think my friends
know the seriousness of
my problem. They look at
me from the outside and
see that I am fine when I
am really in a lot of
physical pain.

I know I should be happy
to be alive, but I'm finding
it harder and harder as my
life goes on. I will try to
have perseverance, to
fight until the end.

I want to go back to school.
I want to walk normally again.
I want to be healthy.

I can't walk and I can't push a wheelchair.
The muscles in my back and leg are weak.
Nerves take time to regenerate.
Too many medical things wrong.

The point that I would freeze time is when
I was eight years old.

I was an innocent and naïve child who had no idea
of the hardships that were to come in my life.
I knew of hardly any evil or sickness, as I lived in
the protected shell of my family's love. I loved going
to school, playing with Barbies and being with my
friends. I could run, skip, dance, skate and swim
with no problems or worries. I had a best friend
who liked me for who I was and who was proud to
have me as a friend. We spent a lot of time together
and knew each other well. My sisters were young
and blameless and they were the centre of my life.
My family was one. At Christmas all my cousins,
aunts, uncles and grandparents would be happy and
never resentful of each other.

My life was almost perfect.

My parents, my sister and I went on a trip to British
Columbia in August of 1987. We had a lot of fun
sightseeing and visiting. One day we went to a
waterslide park. I was so excited. I went up the stairs
to the waterslide with no problems. I was scared but
I knew everything would be all right. As I started on

my way down, my stomach was in my throat.

When I hit the water, my fears were released. I had enjoyed myself and was very content. I was unsuspecting and unaware that my life would never be the same.

We left the waterslide park, never to return. This is the exact moment that I would freeze in my life.

I was a youthful girl who loved life. I had no disease or sickness. I was a small child who just had the time of her life.

I am not sure if I would be the same person as I am today had I actually frozen time at this point. I would not have known the true value of life. I would not have the perspective on life that I have today.

Even though I know deep down that everything happens for a reason, I have yet to figure out why my fate was changed.

I wish I was still a child who was able to live that
normal life.

I am one in a million.

I have stumped a lot of doctors.
They don't know of anyone else with
five spinal cord tumours. No one knows
anything about my illness.

My theory is that doctors only know as
much as they are exposed to. They are
not Gods and don't have all the answers.

There is a picture of me at the age of seven in my
First Communion gown and veil hanging on
the wall in my bedroom.

I was so proud of myself in that attire and felt like a
princess living on the clouds. I was smiling so much
that the photographer told me not to smile so much.
That is the instant my childhood began to vanish
before my eyes.

The picture that is hanging in my room is of a girl
who is happy on the inside but with a straight face
on the outside. Two years later I was diagnosed with
cancer. Every time I look at that picture, I am
reminded of all the facades I have put on in my life.
I always say I am okay or fine but really, I am
confused and angry. I have struggled together with
my family through so much and I try desperately to
come to terms with the obstacles I have faced in
my life.

My facial expression in the portrait expresses the
feelings I experience so often in my life. I was
forced to grow up. Forced to face the possibility of
death and paralysis. Forced to skip playing with
Barbies, going to dances and getting drunk.

Forced to jump into the adult mentality of structure and courage. (Something I am not too sure I have done well with).

Some of the most devastating times in
my life are my clearest memories. Why?
Is it because I haven't dealt with my
feelings about them?

When I was re-diagnosed in grade nine,
I felt a huge void – like a part of me had
been ripped out. Like all my dreams and
aspirations had been taken away from me.

I desperately want to be the person I was in
grade seven and eight. I was the person
who was on my way to achieving the goals
I had set out for myself. Those same
dreams are still in my heart and I know I
will achieve them eventually but it's not the
time I wanted things to happen. I was
supposed to do all these things from the
ages of thirteen to eighteen. Then I was
going to go to university and begin a new
life. Unfortunately, I'm still a baby and need
my mother to help me do everything.

I don't like the way my life has turned out,
but I know I have to take 'one day at a time'
– that's all a person can deal with. I realize
that what has happened to me has made me
a stronger and better person, but I like to
be in control.

When I hear commercials on TV saying, "Plan your future", I get upset because you can plan all you want, but if something is going to ruin your plans you can't do anything about it. You can only accept them and deal with them the best way you can. I believe that society today believes that life will go as planned and never to expect anything less.

TV shows, movies and books usually portray a world that is perfect. Everyone has boyfriends, cars, houses and nice clothes. This portrayal is wrong since there are people starving, homeless and less fortunate.

I wish I could just accept
myself for who I am and for
what I look like.

But in such a superficial society,
anyone who is not tall, thin and
gorgeous is not accepted in the
normal group. I think all I
really want to be is "normal"
again and although I know I
will never be tall, I do want to
be thinner and prettier.

Sometimes I feel like I am ninety and
have wisdom and knowledge that can
help younger people.

I feel a distance between people my
age like I am years older than them.
But I also feel like a little kid who
knows nothing about things and
doesn't understand everything I am
supposed to. For example, I know
nothing about banking, or working and
cry every time I get really angry. I have
been trying to overcome this but it
doesn't seem to be working.

I think I have anger building up in me.
I really don't know who or what I'm
angry at. Am I angry at myself? My
parents? My family? Or just at the
whole world for ruining my plans for
my life?

The Honorary Medal Of Achievement

The next award I would like to present is to two young girls.
These young ladies have showed us that hard work,
perseverance, and the love of dance can help you through
whatever obstacles life may bring. About eight years ago a
group of energetic, beautiful, young dancers performed at the
Kiwanis Festival dressed as bellboys holding little red suitcases
as their props. It was quite odd that that summer two
members of that group became seriously ill. Throughout the
years their devotion to dance was never forgotten. Whatever
physical activity they were able to do, they were back at the
studio dancing in one form or another. These two girls have
shown that the arts play a very important role in everyone's
life, be it music, theatre or dance. I would like to present
Jennifer Smith* and Laura Cotesta with an honourary medal
of achievement. Their love of dance is an inspiration for all.

As I heard Miss Ida's words, the memories started to
flood my mind. My heart began to race. My stomach
was full of butterflies and my eyes were bursting
with tears. I pushed myself up from my seat and
started to limp down the aisle. Everyone's face was a
blur. When I reached the stage, I forced myself up
the stairs. I felt Miss Ida's arms around my shoulders
as she hugged me. She put the shining medal around
my neck. I walked to stand next to the line of
dancers, in the place where I should have been, but

in a costume. I stood there in disbelief, realizing that all my hard work had paid off. At that moment, I came to a conclusion. At the end of every storm there is sunshine and if I kept hoping, praying and fighting against the odds, the sunshine in my life was sure to come.

*Name has been changed to protect privacy.

hope

· · · · · · · · · · · · · · · · · · ·

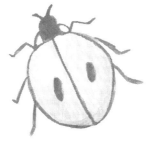

As a seventeen-year-old girl, whose wishes and dreams have been shattered more than once, I am attempting to encourage myself on to a new path in life that will lead me away from disappointment and onto glory.

The road that is chosen for us is sometimes not one we would like to follow but we are sometimes forced on. My life has been full of little side roads that I have been led on, but I am committed to finding the main road again and continuing on with my life.

My primary goal is to be in perfect health
by the age of twenty.

Being healthy in mind, spirit and my physical body is
something that I am presently working very hard at
doing. The fact that I am dependent on others at this
point in my life has motivated me to becoming
physically able to do things for myself. Getting rid of
any tumour, scar-tissue, braces and canes are my
number one priority. By the time I am twenty I wish
to be in perfect health both physically and mentally.

Having a good scholastic career is something that is
also very important to me. I want to graduate high
school with an average of at least 85 and attend a
university in pursuit of a prosperous and fulfilling
future in the field of my choice.

I wish to complete my lifeguarding courses and
continue on in some of my skating levels and
possibly be on the board of directors of a skating
club. Being as smart as I can be in my educational
endeavours is a very important goal for me.

Having the respect of my peers as a mature and
responsible person is of much significance to me.

I feel that being mature and being able to make good decisions is a prominent building block in life. I wish to be a self-confident, independent woman of the 1990's who knows what she wants and how to get it the best way possible.

I want to have friends who like me for who I am and respect me for my determination and hard-work.

Although I may be only seventeen, I know there are many paths to take in life, I am confident that my path of disappointment has come to an end. My road to recovery is going to take a lot of hard work, but my perseverance will help me through. From now until the age of twenty and through the rest of my life, I will try to accomplish the goals of being in perfect health, having a good scholastic career, and being respected by others as a mature and responsible human being.

"Footprints" is my favourite poem because it reminds me of the many times that I have questioned God and asked him for the help and courage to get through the tough times in life. It reassures me that God was there helping me through my hardships and will continue to be there, guiding me through my life. The poem also helps me to remember all the good and exciting times in my life and the enjoyable characteristics of it.

A Skaters Dream

She glides onto the ice,
her dress is so nice.
She takes her position,
with all intuition.

She moves elegantly across the ice,
pushing strong, spinning twice.
Moving so peacefully to the music,
listening carefully to every acoustic.

Skating with strength and grace,
jumping high, flying through space.
Feeling like she's touched the skies,
tears of joy come to her eyes.

Winning gold is her dream.
She smiles as the crowd begins to scream.
Her dreams of glory soaring high,
she curtsies without a sigh.

Her marks come next.
Now this is the test.
Five nine, six point zero.
She feels she's a hero.

Being #1 was her quest,
for now, she knows she is the best.
Now nothing can stand in her way.
All disappointment is far away.

I am a true extension of my mother.

We are like one person and count on each other for support in times of hardship and for strength and courage when trying to overcome obstacles. When I was in the hospital this past May, I hated to see my mom's face when my dad and my sisters were leaving to come home. She wanted to cry; she wanted to run after them and beg them not to leave but could not. I told her it would not be long before we returned home, and that everything would be all right. She believed me.

When I felt down because I could not move my head, neck, back, arms and legs, she gave me the courage by telling me the same words I told her. My mother's never-ending demonstration of her love towards me is something I will treasure in my heart forever. Her love is fulfilling for me and for herself. I believe that she wants to help me and love me wholeheartedly all of the time.

I tell my mother everything. I cannot lie to her or keep things from her. She can tell if I am and I break down and tell her the truth. My mom respects my relationships with my peers and never asks me to reveal their secrets.

I know my mother is wise and knowledgeable because almost every piece of advice she has given me has been the right one. Even when I do not listen and take my own advice, usually ending in a mistake, she is always there to help me.

My mother is my best friend and I know I can count on her whenever I need to. As I am growing older I am realizing more than ever that the saying, mothers know what is best for their children, is absolutely correct.

My mom always tries to guide me on the right path in life. Her life experience prior to my birth and the experiences we have gone through together have made her a strong person whom I admire and look up to. I think that as life is progressing both my mom and I are learning more about ourselves and each other than we thought was imaginable.

For all these reasons, I believe that my mother, Giuseppina Cotesta, truly knows who I am, after all she is my best friend.

My mother has always been by my side, caring and protecting me throughout my many struggles.

Over the past nine years I have undergone five operations to my spine and three doses of radiation therapy. These have all amounted to prolonged hospital stays at the Hospital for Sick Children in Toronto. My mother never left my side. She nursed me back to health and did everything in her power to make sure I received the best medical treatment possible.

She truly understands my feelings and I understand hers. The bond we share is something very special – a rarity that I am proud and honoured to have the chance to experience. My mother usually knows how I feel. She can tell when I am angry or sad and tries to help me through the problem.

I called her from the hospital the other day. I was angry with one of the nurses. My mother could tell by the sound of my voice that something was bothering me. She guessed what it was and gave me advice on how to fix the problem.

Sometimes we will even say the same things, start

the same conversation with different people, wear
the same colours of clothing and pick out the same
things when shopping. The other day, I got dressed
in my black jeans and a white sweater. About ten
minutes later, my mother walked into my room
wearing exactly the same colours as me.

Later on, that same day, my sister asked me, "Laura,
what do you want for lunch?" I replied, "I feel like
having Kraft Dinner." When my mom returned
home my sister asked my mom the same question.
Sure enough, my mom said, "I feel like having Kraft
Dinner."

These occurrences are happening so often I think I
am turning into her. I sometimes think we are the
same person. We react the same in certain situations
and we are both perfectionists.

I have learned excellent values from my family.

The most important values I have learned are: determination, courage and strength.

My family has gone through many hard times, most of which deal with my illness. Throughout everything, I think I have been a strong person who is determined to achieve her goals. I don't think I would have been able to jump all the hurdles without the love and support of my parents. Their courage and perseverance inspire me.

I truly believe my family is loving and stable and that they have taught me how to be determined, courageous and strong.

I believe people die when they are at peace
with themselves and when they have
done their job on earth.

I believe my grandfather died in peace. His brother
and sisters were to arrive from Italy the day after my
grandfather was brought to emergency. He had
stopped breathing and probably should have died
then. He was very sick and was hooked up to
respirators and ventilators. Miraculously, the next
day he was a lot better and even stood up.

After he visited with his sisters and brother, I never
saw my grandfather happier. That day I told my
grandfather I loved him and he said it back. I know
that the moment he said, "I love you too," is
probably one of the most peaceful and happiest
moments of my life. During the night he died.
His last words were, "Tell Laura I love her."

I truly believed he wanted to see his brother and
sisters so he could die happy and in peace. His death
was a shock, although we knew it was bound to
happen. As I think back, I think it happened at the
perfect time. I miss my grandfather tremendously,
but I am at peace, for I know he died happy.

As I looked at my Nonno laying in the casket with his arms across his chest, I realized how much I would miss his tender and fragile touch.

I was glad that I had told him I loved him a few days before. I had no regrets or worries. My heart was filled up with his love and caring.

Never again will I feel the peace and sorrow and mixed emotions I felt that day. The whole experience taught me that if you love and respect people while they are alive, they will respect you back by watching over you in heaven.

My Nonno's last words were, "Don't forget to tell Laura that I love her." I will hold those words dear to my heart forever.

I wonder why my grandfather's funeral is such a major memory of my life. Is it because it taught me about death and how to accept it? If I die, I want to die happy. I believe my Nonno did. His death taught me to better accept it and not to be so afraid of death.

Society today seems to have a hard time dealing with death. I really have no idea why, but I suspect it is because our faith in higher powers has been altered by media images and false interpretations that people have made.

I believe in God and that He controls what happens in life. I can't say that I really understand why He is making me go through what I am experiencing. As a matter of fact, I am a bit angry at Him. I never did anything wrong as a child and I don't think I deserve all the pain and suffering I am going through.

I think about this often. There must be a reason for it all. Is it so I will teach others? Is it so I will learn more about myself? Or is a combination of both? Will it all be over once I have learned everything about myself?

Am I on a journey of self-discovery?

Was it meant for me to find the faults within myself, and rediscover who I truly am? I know I am not the same person I was years ago. I have changed and become stronger in character and more outspoken. Sometimes I wonder if this change in me has actually been for the better.

I want desperately to be the person I was before I got sick; I want to be that healthy eight-year-old who skated, danced and swam. I want to live a normal life and have a real group of friends that come over to my house and do everything with me and who I feel is like my family. I resent not getting the chance to do this. I wonder what my life would be like if I had never gotten sick. I guess that is only natural.

Maybe all of this is happening to me so I learn to love myself just the way I am. Although this is probably true, I can't seem to bring myself to do it. I always care about what others are thinking of me and I desperately seek approval and acceptance into my peer group. I seem to have a problem because the people who are my friends and know my history

so well, seem to be afraid of me and do not know
what to say to me. I really don't know what to say to
them either.

I feel so different and secluded. I feel that I am in a world of my own, a world longing to fit into society again.

I want to be able to go out and not have to worry about the number of steps or cleaning my wheels before I go into someone's house. I want to jump around and express myself at a party and get into trouble for being late. I want to be able to hop into the car and drive away and I want to be totally independent and free to choose and make decisions that don't always depend on my health.

I want so desperately to help everyone. Perhaps this is why I am such a worrier. But why do I find it so hard to help myself? Is it because I just want to avoid what is happening to me? Or is it just part of my nature?

I hope that one day
everything will just click for
me. That I will find out the
truth about myself and be at
peace with life. I hope this
happens soon and many
years before I die, so that I
can learn my true identity
and accept myself for who I
am. I think that this would
be the greatest feeling
although it will probably
include suffering. Then and
only then, will I be able to
fully comprehend and
understand the impact that I
have made on others and if I
truly am the good person I
think myself to be.

I want to die in peace and gradually so I can live each day to the fullest. If I die suddenly I think I would be stripped of the opportunity to say everything I wanted to say to the people I loved the most.

I think my greatest fear in life would be to die suddenly and not have the opportunity to redeem myself and ask for forgiveness for all my wrong doings in life. After all, I do want to end up as an angel in heaven with my grandfather and the many other people I love, for heaven is the only place of true tranquility and peace.

The quality of self-knowledge is the greatest quality to have in life. Once you have obtained it, you either accept it and live in peace, or ignore it and live in blindness.

I hope I will learn to see the world more clearly so that the chapter of my life that I am living right now will be behind me so I can continue in a new life of happiness and peace. I don't really know if this is possible in the society we live in today, but one can dream – that is something I will always do.

I like telling my story. I actually want to write a book about it. I feel like I am letting go of my emotions and freeing my soul.

I don't want people to believe that what has happened to me was my fault. When I tell people my story, I hope they will better understand and appreciate me for who I am.

I think though, sometimes I scare people away. They don't know what to say or do when they are around me, so they avoid me. This is one of the hardest things for me to deal with.

Just because I had cancer doesn't mean I am less of a person. In fact, I think I am a better person from it.

I can't quite feel sympathy for my friends who don't call, don't visit and don't try to talk to me. I don't know why they are shutting me out. I feel normal and look normal except for the wheelchair I am sitting in. I often struggle with myself and try to convince myself that everyone sees me, not the chair. I am a person who has always cared about what I look like and what others think of me. This is why I am finding it so difficult to go through these hard times in my life with hardly any peer support.

I know people care about me but sometimes I wish they would show it more often.

My friends are already planning who they are going to semi and grad with and what they are going to wear. I don't care about boys, going to parties, getting drunk and the other things they care about. I can't say I don't think about those things too, but they are not my focus.

I consider myself lucky to be alive
and doing well when I see what other
things people are going through.

I realize that I can still think straight
(although sometimes I wonder) and
can sit in a class with people my age
and still keep up.

I always try hard and have a drive in
me that won't let me give up until I get
what I want – TO BE NORMAL.

I consider myself lucky to have such a supportive family who loves me. I guess I am lucky in a lot of ways but I will never be happy because I am constantly striving for more.

I don't think I give myself the credit I deserve but I sometimes feel like the walls are coming down on me and I expect too many things from myself. I want to get better now, do well in English class (by getting caught up), I want to help out in the school. But I can't. I get tired fast and think that I am letting myself and others down by not doing everything I know. I have to calm down and take things slowly, but my patience is running out.

On the last day I was at the hospital, my roommate asked me to sign her autograph book. I sought to give her courage and strength so I wrote my motto, "If you keep hoping and praying for the sunshine, the sunshine is sure to come." I wrote some other things like "keep smiling" and "always try your best". I gave her the book back. As she read it, I could tell by her face there was something wrong. She didn't understand what I wrote.

Then it dawned on me; she was kicked out of school twice and only had four credits and she was seventeen. The girl never got a chance to learn. How lucky am I to be so aware and informed by my education and eagerness to learn.

I believe I have learned how to look within
myself and see myself differently than before.
I am indeed a strong person with the
determination to succeed in life.

I have surrendered to my wheelchair.

Last year I struggled a lot. My strength was deteriorating and I was getting bad pain in my shoulders, but I persisted.

They told me to sit in a wheelchair, they told me it would make my life easier. But I wouldn't give in. I thought that if I sat in a wheelchair while I could still walk, I would be giving up. Now that it is my only mode of indoor transportation, I realize if I would have given in, it would have made the last months before my fifth diagnosis a little more bearable.

I have had to swallow my pride and let go of my fears to make it through these last few months.

Being in a wheelchair, I see how society does not want to accept people for who they are, but rather for who they want them to be.

Some people don't even acknowledge your persistence. Is our society so afraid of sickness and abnormalities that it can't even see how hard we, the ones who are suffering, are trying?

I am determined to get better. I will once again be a "normal" person who can dance, skate and swim. I have been juggling my schooling and my health for the past four years. I feel like all my hard work has taken me here.

I don't even think people my age realize everything I am going through. Why can't they accept me for who I am now? Why can't I accept myself for who I am?

Do I need someone to tell me perseverance and courage is an inspiration to them? I think so. I think I am longing for this deep inside my soul. I want to be an inspiration to others. I want to be recognized and rewarded for my hard work by my peers.

I actually may be an inspiration to others without knowing it.

Doctors don't know why I can walk with braces or do the things I do.

They are amazed at how someone with so little muscles can do so much. One doctor even called me a "little superhero". Why is this not enough for me? Why do I always strive for more? What is inside of me that is causing this?

Am I who I am because of my sickness? What would I be if I had never gotten sick? I would be "normal." Now, is that really what I want to be, or is it just a desire instilled in me through society? I know deep down I will never be normal, but my desire still burns within me.

I believe my sickness is a voyage.

A voyage to find a deeper understanding and acceptance of myself as well as a journey to teach others about my illness. Honestly, I feel like I am teaching the medical profession about determination and the drive to achieve goals.

When your health is in jeopardy you don't feel like yourself, there is so much you want to do and can't. Then, you truly realize the meaning of life and cherish it.

My cancer came back after six years.

One day I was figure skating and the next
I couldn't even walk.

One day my sisters were average figure skaters
and the next they were Sudbury Regional
Champions and Northern Ontario Sectional
Champions.

One day there is peace and the next there is war.

Why does life have to be this way? In many
respects, it is a good thing but in other ways it is
not. It is good because it adds flavour and variety
to life but is bad because disappointments come
too quickly. There really is no resolution to this
except to take life day by day.

Right now, I am one in a million people who has had an ependymoma spinal cord tumour. The fact that it has returned five times is even more unbelievable. Because of my rare type of tumour, I don't think a cure will be found in time to save my life from deteriorating.

I know that there are probably still some cancer cells floating inside of me. I don't know where they are or when they will come back, but I know they are there. I have a feeling that this is the last time I will get sick for a long time to come. I have this sneaky feeling though, that one day when I am an old lady, sitting on the porch in my rocking chair, I will feel them come alive for the last time, so they can take me to the gates of truth.

What Is Love?

Like a bridge, love joins people together,
in good times, and bad, and in any kind of weather.
Through kindness and sorrow,
it sees you through until tomorrow.

Love is like a candle that burns bright,
in times of darkness and times of light.
With it's never ending warmth by your side,
love is something you can't hide.

Love is like a medical drug,
that cures you when times are smug.
When love's around and things are down,
you just have to smile, and never frown.

Love is like a long journey,
through ups and downs it can be blurry.
Love can't be touched or seen,
it is truly just part of being.

Love is beautiful, love is kind,
love isn't something of the mind.
It can't be written on a chart,
it can only be felt deep down in your heart.

As one grows older,
life gets more complex and difficult.

No one is perfect and we all have our own faults
and things we don't really like about ourselves.
When life gets hard, or the people we love are in
danger, we often think back to the past. We
remember the good times and bad times and wish
we could go back and live the times of happiness
again.

In our society today, there are many fears which are
instilled into us. I believe that one of society's
greatest fears is death. But why? Is death not a part
of life that everyone must encounter and face? Is
death not something we are supposed to find
comfort in?

Is it better to die with your eyes open to reality than
die in falsehood? This is a choice you must make on
your own.

Nothing is more beautiful than to see yourself dying.

In order for you to truly understand the reality of this statement you must go through a journey of self-discovery which leads to the acceptance of death. This journey consists of the following five steps:

1. Know yourself and see the world clearly.

2. Accept death as a part of life.

3. Embrace the experience of dying.

4. Find the true meaning in death.

5. Know what is essential and important in living-relationships, family, friends, honesty and trust.

My inspiration comes from within myself and the
knowledge of who I really am has
helped me along the way.

I have come to terms with this wheelchair and that
society doesn't like people who are different. After
being diagnosed with cancer five times, I have been
through many hardships which have caused me to
look within myself and discover who I truly am. I
have accepted my faults and that I am a person who
longs for acceptance and who wants desperately to
be normal again. I believe I have come to my
acceptance of death by confronting my fear of it.

Through everything, I have learned that the most
important people in life are my Mom and Dad, my
sisters, my grandparents and my aunts. I have
learned that family will always be there for you and
never let you down in times of need.

I have also learned that it doesn't matter how hard I
try, I can only change myself to be an inspiration to
others. I know I will walk again and I know I will be
successful in life, after all I have been given the
quality of self-knowledge (and the opportunity to
see my own death before it happens).

I hope that what you have learned is that going through hardships only makes you a stronger person. If you accept what happens and live each day to the fullest, you can find true value in life and accept yourself for who you are.

Death is a part of life that everyone must encounter and face. Confronting death or coming close to it helps one to accept it as a part of life.

One must go through a journey of self-discovery in which the quality of self-knowledge is rooted within oneself. Once the ability to see the world clearly is established, one can move on and accept death as a part of life. Then by embracing the experience of dying, one can find the genuine meaning of life.

Truly accepting death and life's experiences leads to the knowledge of what is important and essential in living: the qualities of love, honesty and trust. As well, the significance of relationships, family and friends in life becomes cvidcnt.

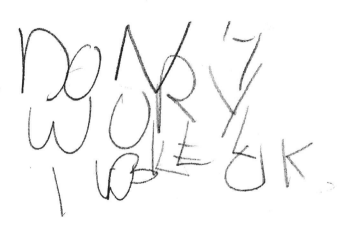

"Don't worry I will be ok."
One of Laura Cotesta's handwritten messages to
family and friends during her final days in hospital.

AFTERWARD

* * * * * * * * * * * * * * * *

I wasn't even one year old when my sister was first diagnosed with cancer and so I don't remember very much about that time and definitely did not truly understand what my sister and parents were going through. What I do remember, is that family was important to Laura. She was our older sister who liked to boss us around. But, she also protected us and was like our second mom.

Our family routine was different than those around me, but I honestly didn't think twice about it. We'd get in the car on Friday, with meals prepared by our Nonna and aunts, and drive to see Laura and my mom in Toronto. We would eat in the cafeteria, explore downtown Toronto with Laura, do arts and crafts together, then come back on Sunday and go back to school, skating and dancing. It was our routine.

I remember feeling comforted that Laura was in such good hands with the experts at SickKids. Laura always had a smile on her face, never looked like she was suffering and seemed to be having fun with the nurses, doctors and other patients. She was surrounded by people who cared and empathized with what she was going through.

When Laura wasn't in Toronto, life back home meant helping her up the stairs, doing her exercises and physio together – and pestering her while she was doing her homework. Family always remained number one. Dinner together was a must, no matter how busy anyone was. She was at every skating competition and would often be the one cheering the loudest. She wanted to make sure I knew she was there for me. Laura was my biggest fan.

The last time we were in Toronto with Laura was surreal. Laura and my mom were at an appointment while Melissa, my dad and I went shopping. My mom called to tell us that Laura had had a seizure and was being rushed to SickKids. We followed the ambulance, speeding down the 401 like we were in a race. That day, we received the news that Laura had twelve tumours in her brain and there wasn't anything more doctors could do for her; it was too

dangerous and too late to operate. She was given
one month to live. Laura promised us, "I'm going to
get through this."

My mom and sister didn't want to sit around and
wait for her to deteriorate, so they decided to travel
to Mexico to try an alternative treatment. When
Laura returned home, she continued going to school
so she could graduate with her classmates. However,
my sister was getting significantly weaker. Our living
room soon became a hospital room and nurses were
constantly coming in and out of the house.
Somehow, Laura made it to graduation, trying so
hard to smile but for the first time, I could see the
pain in her eyes. I could see that she was suffering
and she would say she just "wanted to go home," to
a place where there was no more pain and where the
sun would shine every day.

But in true Laura style, her last breath in this
world was well thought out. After being rushed to
the ICU and being told she probably wouldn't make
it through the night, Laura miraculously woke up.
She was on a respirator and wanted so badly to
speak but couldn't. Instead, she handwrote messages
on paper. She needed to tell everyone who meant
something to her, thank-you and goodbye. Laura
was surrounded by those whom she loved most –
the waiting room was packed with friends and

family. Later that night, she started breathing on her own again and was moved to another floor. None of us wanted to leave, but my mom insisted that Laura just needed to rest. That night, when she was all alone with just my mom - her rock, strength and trust - she took her last breath.

So, what happened after that? Well, life is kind of a blur. Anyone who has lost someone close to them will understand what I mean. I was eleven, had lost my oldest sister and had no clue how to help my parents or Melissa deal with this. We all had heavy hearts but tried to be strong for one another and to continue on with life. My mom and dad made sure that Melissa and I were still involved in skating and dancing and that we were still working hard at school. We went through the motions and just tried to make sense of what we had just been through and how we were going to move on without Laura. Life wasn't the same. None of us were the same.

Still, my memories of Laura are positive and full of life. The picture I have of her in my head is one where she has a big smile on her face, one that could light up a room. I share her love and commitment to family, and so moved home after completing university and started my teaching career in Sudbury. Her strength and courage throughout all her difficulties guided me through challenges I've encountered. Her positive outlook on life is embedded in me and I try to live looking at the bright side of things because of her, every day of my life. Her need to help others has guided me in my teaching career and my future goals.

Laura was a gift, someone truly special. She taught most people she met something and has managed to continue teaching those who learn about her story. Laura left a lasting impression, even impacted her friends' future life choices. She has helped them to become better people, helped them to empathize and understand the struggles of others.

Cancer affects so many people. And when it happens to you, it feels like you and your family are the only ones in the struggle. You feel isolated, alone and scared. The purpose of this book is to remind you that you are not alone. You're not alone because someone else has lived through the same or similar experience. Whether you are the one fighting cancer, or the parent, sibling, friend, or an extended family member, you are not alone in feeling the way you do; everyone is hurting. Try to talk about your feelings and I promise, you will feel better. The sun will shine, even for a little.

- DANIELA COTESTA

Many of us are afraid of death. I think it's because we don't want to leave without doing everything we had hoped to do. We don't want to leave with regrets. We want to leave our mark.

Laura wasn't afraid. If there's one thing this book shows, it is that one young woman, with an enormous spirit, and a clear faithful vision can make her mark.

Laura feared needles, breaking the rules, and upsetting my parents, but she was never afraid of what lay ahead. It's pretty surreal when I look back. In eighteen years of life, my sister was able to accomplish more than most of us do in a lifetime. She was eloquent, she listened, and she never complained. Laura taught us through her time on earth and continues to teach us through her words.

Laura was courageous and she helped others be courageous too. In turn, she gave my mom the courage to travel, explore, investigate and be an advocate for her daughter. I remember watching the two of them walking together out of the hospital, after Laura had received treatment minutes before, into what we believed were the dangerous streets of Toronto. They were on their way to shop for matching dresses for the three of us for the next celebration. With Laura's hand in hers, my mom wasn't afraid. My mom could face anything thanks to Laura's own courage.

Some memories of Laura and our journey as a family remain vivid while others have faded. I remember hearing the word "cancer" and not grasping what was happening. By the age of ten Laura knew what was important. She focused on her family and she had a deep connection with her passion and purpose. As a child, she knew how to describe what she was feeling; she knew how to relate to anyone, both young and old, and she had an infectious smile that never showed her sadness. Her eyes were so deep and filled with stories. She was so wise and focused.

She listened, she fought.

I hated so much of what happened to my sister and our family. This kind of thing changes people. I hated being in hospitals, I hated the smell of the rooms, I hated that we had to pack food and eat out of thermoses. To this day, I can't eat pasta or soup out of a thermos. I hated staying in hotels, and sharing a bed, or sleeping on the floor. I hated having to depend on other people to drive me around. Although I was well taken care of, I learned independence at a young age.

I was upset about not being able to go out with my friends. Meanwhile Laura was stuck at home, needing assistance just to do the simplest things like going to the washroom. I remember her feeling like her independence and dignity were lost, but she never lost sight of the big picture. I would ask her all the time, "Why do you even care about school?" It was such hard work for her, more difficult than any of us could ever imagine. In high school we don't even want to go to class when we have a pimple, let alone when we need leg braces or a wheelchair just to get around. Laura somehow knew that her story was about awareness, about life, about love and about a movement.

You do not forget or recover from losses so great. You aspire to move forward but carry this loss with you. My family did remarkably well, and that is all because of Laura. Somehow, even though she was the child, she protected each and every one of us from so much. As a child this girl had more insight and perspective than most of us have in adulthood. She listened. She knew what we needed and she made sure she did everything in her power to give it to us.

What I didn't realize back then was how lucky I was to have such a presence in my life. All of these years later, she still guides my every decision. As her sister, I am blessed to have this force and experience to guide me through my life. Her life gives me perspective. Her life and these stories are what guide me when things are not going the way I had hoped. She helps me focus on the big picture, to understand the fragility of life, to accept that sometimes we have no control, to understand the medical field can't save us all and to believe in a power beyond us.

I realize there is nothing unique about a child succumbing to cancer and leaving an impact on her family. But I also realize that this girl was not just a child, she was a ray of sunshine spreading the word to ensure that whoever is chosen next to fight this battle has every chance to enjoy the small things in life, spend as much time as they can with the people they love, and most of all not live in fear of death. Every day is a gift.

This is a story that goes beyond my memories. It reaches the soul. The universe was guiding Laura and she was paying attention. Now it's time to reflect on the miracle of it all.

- MELISSA COTESTA

"Don't forget me."
One of Laura Cotesta's handwritten messages to
family and friends during her final days in hospital.

"Laura's impact on the students of Lockerby Composite School is one that has been enduring. Through the Kids Caring for Kids Remembering Laura Cotesta Cancer Drive, she reminds us to be courageous, to persevere and to spread kindness. I believe that her words and actions remind our students to never lose hope and to never give up. Twenty years later, her message is still delivered to new groups of adolescents who are searching for role models. I know that they find one in Laura Cotesta. The special energy in our building the night of the Cancer Drive is Laura's legacy."

- JENNIFER PELOSO, Teacher, Lockerby Composite School

Editor's note: As of 2018, the Kids Caring for Kids Remembering Laura Cotesta Cancer Drive raised close to $1 million for the Northern Cancer Foundation and pediatric cancer care in Northern Ontario.

ACKNOWLEDGEMENTS

Special thanks to my family, Melissa, Daniela and Giulio for their continued patience and guidance. They provided me with the space and support to see this project through.

I imagine Laura would like to thank her family as well, for their selflessness and understanding in her own journey. To her sisters for sharing such a wonderful childhood together. There is a bond between sisters that is immeasurable.

Laura would want me to thank her friends, teachers, guidance counsellors and educational workers who listened and showed compassion. Also, the medical community – doctors, nurses, occupational therapists, physiotherapists – for taking good care of her on earth.

139

You were all instrumental in helping Laura live a fulfilled life. Our family is forever grateful to everyone.

I would like to acknowledge those who contributed to the creation of this book.

To Laura Stradiotto for reviewing hundreds of pages of Laura's journals, essays and school work and ensuring her voice remained authentic, to Cristina Borgogelli for the cover illustration and Prajna Gandhi for designing the book – we thank you from the bottom of our hearts.

Thank you to Ronda Lenti for believing in Laura, having faith in her words and working tirelessly to bring this book to reality and for compiling and organizing the history of Lockerby Composite School's Kids Caring for Kids Remembering Laura Cotesta Cancer Drive. To Roberto Bagnato for helping to organize and maintain the website so that Laura's story and the success of Lockerby's Cancer Drive can be shared with people worldwide.

And to all the wonderful people who submitted their heartfelt memories; for remembering Laura in a positive way and her impact on our lives, you have ensured that the sun continues to shine today.

I applaud you for all your love, your compassion and your smiles.

- PINA COTESTA